MEDITERRANEAN DIET VEGETARIAN RECIPES FOR TYPE 1 DIABETES

30 Days of Delicious Mediterranean Vegetarian Meals for Blood Sugar Balance

T. John

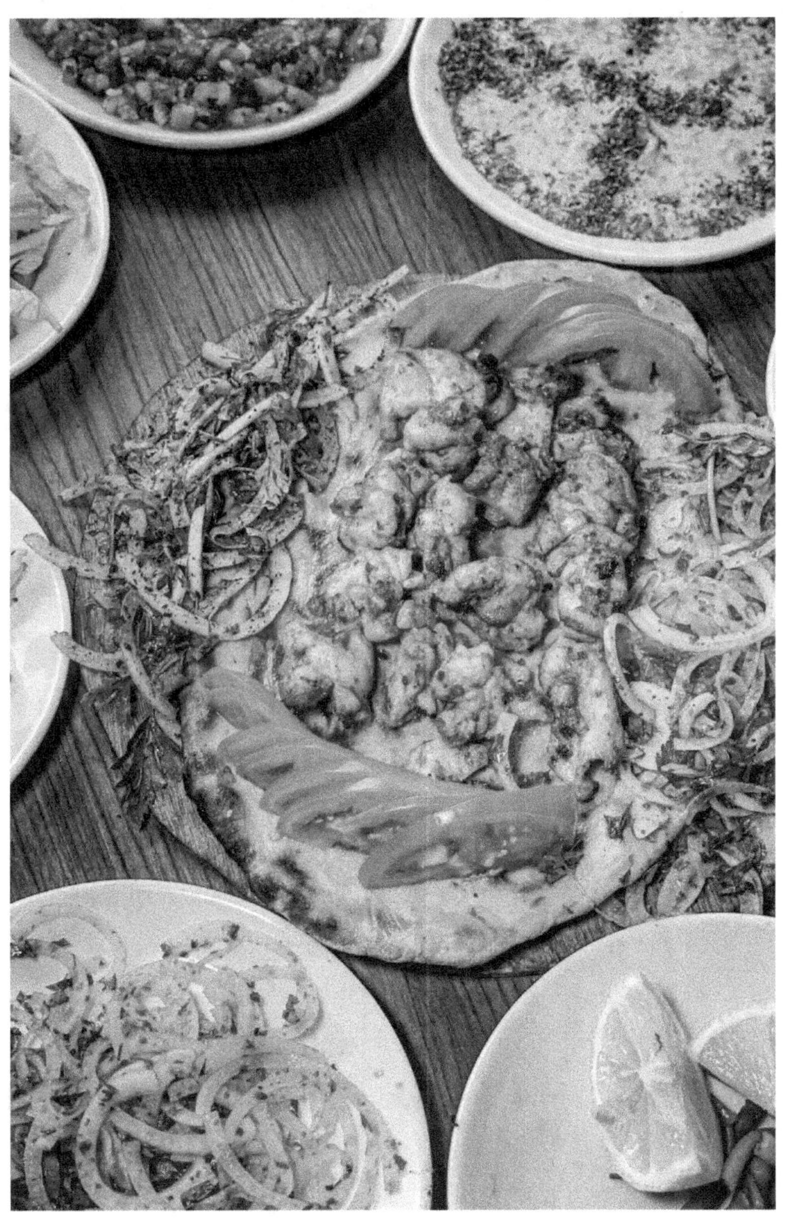

TABLE OF CONTENTS

INTRODUCTION

F orget fads and quick fixes – let's embark on a vibrant culinary journey where taste tangoes with health. We'll unravel the Mediterranean Diet, explore the vibrant world of vegetarianism, and discover how food can become a powerful ally in managing Type 1 Diabetes.

The Mediterranean Diet

Imagine plates overflowing with fresh, sun-drenched ingredients. Picture olive oil glistening on crisp salads, plump olives dotting rustic bread, and fish bathed in fragrant herbs. This isn't just a meal; it's the Mediterranean Diet, an ode to deliciousness and well-being.

This isn't a rigid script, but a flexible melody. Think bountiful vegetables and fruits, singing in harmony with whole grains and legumes. Extra virgin olive oil, the conductor, orchestrates the rhythm, while herbs and spices add a vibrant melody. Don't forget fatty fish, like tuna and salmon, occasionally gracing the stage. And what's a symphony without wine? Enjoy a moderate glass in good company, adding a touch of cheer.

This vibrant medley isn't just a culinary delight; it's a health powerhouse. Research whispers sweet nothings about reduced risk of heart disease, diabetes, and even dementia. It's a symphony for your body, playing a tune of well-being.

Embracing Plant-Powered Plates

But some prefer a different beat. Enter the Veggie Revolution, a movement where vegetables take center stage. From succulent stir-fries to creamy curries, plant-based plates paint a canvas of flavor and health.

This isn't just about avoiding meat; it's about embracing a bounty of possibilities. Think protein-packed lentils and beans, dancing with roasted vegetables in a rainbow of colors. Tofu and tempeh, the understudies, can take on any flavor, while fresh herbs and spices add a touch of drama.

And the benefits? They're not shy. Lower cholesterol, better blood sugar control, and a reduced risk of chronic diseases join the chorus of praise. It's a movement for a healthier you, a revolution on your plate.

Food as Medicine for Type 1 Diabetes

For those diagnosed with Type 1 Diabetes, food isn't just fuel; it's a tool. Understanding carbohydrates, the sugar bandits hiding in food, becomes crucial. But this isn't a battle; it's a dance.

Planning meals becomes a strategic ballet. Whole grains, like brown rice and quinoa, offer slow-burning energy, while fruits and vegetables add vitamins and fiber without spiking blood sugar. Lean protein keeps you feeling full, and healthy fats, like those found in avocado and nuts, add a touch of richness.

But remember, this dance has no fixed steps. Individual needs vary, and a registered dietitian becomes your choreographer, helping you design a personalized routine. With knowledge as your guide and delicious food as your fuel, you can manage Type 1 Diabetes and keep it off your toes.

So, dear reader, whether you're drawn to the Mediterranean melody, the Veggie Revolution's beat, or the mindful dance of managing Type 1 Diabetes, remember: food is more than just sustenance. It's a story waiting to be told, a symphony to be savored, and a powerful tool for health and well-being. Take a bite, embrace the flavor, and discover the transformative power of a mindful, delicious diet.

Chapter 1: 30 Day Meal Plan

Week 1:

Day 1:

- Breakfast: Mediterranean Scrambled Tofu
- Lunch: Lentil and Vegetable Salad
- Dinner: Mediterranean Stuffed Zucchini Boats
- Snack: Hummus with Veggie Sticks
- Dessert: Greek Yogurt with Honey and Nuts

Day 2:

- Breakfast: Spinach and Feta Omelette
- Lunch: Greek Salad Wrap
- Dinner: Baked Eggplant Parmesan
- Snack: Mediterranean Bruschetta
- Dessert: Mixed Berry Sorbet

Day 3:

- Breakfast: Quinoa Breakfast Bowl
- Lunch: Mediterranean Quinoa Bowl
- Dinner: Lemon Garlic Orzo with Roasted Vegetables

- Snack: Olive and Artichoke Tapenade
- Dessert: Almond Flour Orange Cake

Day 4:

- Breakfast: Greek Yogurt Parfait
- Lunch: Stuffed Bell Peppers with Couscous
- Dinner: Artichoke and Sundried Tomato Risotto
- Snack: Greek Yogurt Dip with Cucumber
- Dessert: Chocolate-Dipped Strawberries

Day 5:

- Breakfast: Avocado Toast with Cherry Tomatoes
- Lunch: Caprese Salad with Balsamic Glaze
- Dinner: Quinoa-Stuffed Bell Peppers
- Snack: Roasted Red Pepper and Feta Dip
- Dessert: Pistachio and Fig Energy Bars

Day 6:

- Breakfast: Chickpea Flour Pancakes
- Lunch: Chickpea and Spinach Stew
- Dinner: Spaghetti Aglio e Olio with Cherry Tomatoes

- Snack: Stuffed Grape Leaves with Tzatziki
- Dessert: Mediterranean Fruit Salad

Day 7:

- Breakfast: Mediterranean Veggie Frittata
- Lunch: Roasted Vegetable and Hummus Wrap
- Dinner: Sweet Potato and Chickpea Tagine
- Snack: Spicy Chickpea Roast
- Dessert: Olive Oil and Lemon Cake

Week 2:

Day 8:

- Breakfast: Zucchini and Tomato Breakfast Casserole
- Lunch: Tomato and Basil Bruschetta
- Dinner: Mediterranean Lentil Soup
- Snack: Sundried Tomato and White Bean Dip
- Dessert: Date and Nut Balls

Day 9:

- Breakfast: Chia Seed Pudding with Berries
- Lunch: Mediterranean Chickpea Salad
- Dinner: Grilled Portobello Mushrooms with Polenta

- Snack: Greek Spanakopita Bites
- Dessert: Baklava-Inspired Yogurt Parfait

Day 10:

- Breakfast: Whole Grain Muesli with Nuts and Dried Fruits
- Lunch: Eggplant and Mozzarella Panini
- Dinner: Ratatouille with Herbed Couscous
- Snack: Roasted Garlic and White Bean Hummus
- Dessert: Roasted Peach with Cinnamon

Day 11:

- Breakfast: Eggplant and Mozzarella Breakfast Sandwich
- Lunch: Spinach and Feta Stuffed Mushrooms
- Dinner: Spinach and Feta Stuffed Chicken Breast
- Snack: Mediterranean Stuffed Mushrooms
- Dessert: Lemon Sorbet with Mint

Day 12:

- Breakfast: Bulgur Porridge with Pistachios
- Lunch: Cucumber and Avocado Sushi Rolls

- Dinner: Pesto Pasta with Cherry Tomatoes
- Snack: Pistachio and Cranberry Energy Bites
- Dessert: Watermelon and Mint Granita

Day 13:

- Breakfast: Sweet Potato and Black Bean Hash
- Lunch: Farro and Roasted Vegetable Bowl
- Dinner: Mediterranean Baked Cod
- Snack: Baked Zucchini Fries
- Dessert: Chia Seed Pudding with Pistachios and Dates

Day 14:

- Breakfast: Mediterranean-style Shakshuka
- Lunch: Mediterranean Pita Sandwich
- Dinner: Zoodles with Tomato and Basil Sauce
- Snack: Avocado and Tomato Salsa
- Dessert: Orange and Walnut Biscotti

Week 3:

Day 15:

- Breakfast: Fig and Almond Tart

- Lunch: Cauliflower and Chickpea Curry
- Dinner: Vegan Paella
- Snack: Caprese Skewers
- Dessert: Greek Yogurt with Honey and Nuts

Day 16:

- Breakfast: Mediterranean Scrambled Tofu
- Lunch: Lentil and Vegetable Salad
- Dinner: Mediterranean Stuffed Zucchini Boats
- Snack: Hummus with Veggie Sticks
- Dessert: Mixed Berry Sorbet

Day 17:

- Breakfast: Spinach and Feta Omelette
- Lunch: Greek Salad Wrap
- Dinner: Baked Eggplant Parmesan
- Snack: Mediterranean Bruschetta
- Dessert: Almond Flour Orange Cake

Day 18:

- Breakfast: Quinoa Breakfast Bowl
- Lunch: Mediterranean Quinoa Bowl

- Dinner: Lemon Garlic Orzo with Roasted Vegetables
- Snack: Olive and Artichoke Tapenade
- Dessert: Chocolate-Dipped Strawberries

Day 19:

- Breakfast: Greek Yogurt Parfait
- Lunch: Stuffed Bell Peppers with Couscous
- Dinner: Artichoke and Sundried Tomato Risotto
- Snack: Greek Yogurt Dip with Cucumber
- Dessert: Pistachio and Fig Energy Bars

Day 20:

- Breakfast: Avocado Toast with Cherry Tomatoes
- Lunch: Caprese Salad with Balsamic Glaze
- Dinner: Quinoa-Stuffed Bell Peppers
- Snack: Roasted Red Pepper and Feta Dip
- Dessert: Mediterranean Fruit Salad

Day 21:

- Breakfast: Chickpea Flour Pancakes
- Lunch: Chickpea and Spinach Stew

- Dinner: Spaghetti Aglio e Olio with Cherry Tomatoes
- Snack: Stuffed Grape Leaves with Tzatziki
- Dessert: Olive Oil and Lemon Cake

Week 4

Day 22:

- Breakfast: Zucchini and Tomato Breakfast Casserole
- Lunch: Tomato and Basil Bruschetta
- Dinner: Mediterranean Lentil Soup
- Snack: Sundried Tomato and White Bean Dip
- Dessert: Date and Nut Balls

Day 23:

- Breakfast: Chia Seed Pudding with Berries
- Lunch: Mediterranean Chickpea Salad
- Dinner: Grilled Portobello Mushrooms with Polenta
- Snack: Greek Spanakopita Bites
- Dessert: Baklava-Inspired Yogurt Parfait

Day 24:

- Breakfast: Whole Grain Muesli with Nuts and Dried Fruits
- Lunch: Eggplant and Mozzarella Panini
- Dinner: Ratatouille with Herbed Couscous
- Snack: Roasted Garlic and White Bean Hummus
- Dessert: Roasted Peach with Cinnamon

Day 25:

- Breakfast: Eggplant and Mozzarella Breakfast Sandwich
- Lunch: Spinach and Feta Stuffed Mushrooms
- Dinner: Spinach and Feta Stuffed Chicken Breast
- Snack: Mediterranean Stuffed Mushrooms
- Dessert: Lemon Sorbet with Mint

Day 26:

- Breakfast: Bulgur Porridge with Pistachios
- Lunch: Cucumber and Avocado Sushi Rolls
- Dinner: Pesto Pasta with Cherry Tomatoes
- Snack: Pistachio and Cranberry Energy Bites
- Dessert: Watermelon and Mint Granita

Day 27:

- Breakfast: Sweet Potato and Black Bean Hash
- Lunch: Farro and Roasted Vegetable Bowl
- Dinner: Mediterranean Baked Cod
- Snack: Baked Zucchini Fries
- Dessert: Chia Seed Pudding with Pistachios and Dates

Day 28:

- Breakfast: Mediterranean-style Shakshuka
- Lunch: Mediterranean Pita Sandwich
- Dinner: Zoodles with Tomato and Basil Sauce
- Snack: Avocado and Tomato Salsa
- Dessert: Orange and Walnut Biscotti

Day 29:

- Breakfast: Fig and Almond Tart
- Lunch: Cauliflower and Chickpea Curry
- Dinner: Vegan Paella
- Snack: Caprese Skewers
- Dessert: Greek Yogurt with Honey and Nuts

Day 30:

- Breakfast: Mediterranean Scrambled Tofu
- Lunch: Lentil and Vegetable Salad
- Dinner: Mediterranean Stuffed Zucchini Boats
- Snack: Hummus with Veggie Sticks
- Dessert: Mixed Berry Sorbet

Chapter 2: Breakfast Recipes

These recipes not only tantalize your taste buds but also align with a vegetarian approach, perfect for those managing Type 1 Diabetes. Each dish is carefully curated to bring you a burst of flavors while considering the nutritional values crucial for a balanced diet.

Mediterranean Scrambled Tofu

Ingredients:

- 1 cup firm tofu, crumbled
- 2 tbsp olive oil
- 1/4 cup cherry tomatoes, halved
- 1/4 cup Kalamata olives, sliced
- 1/4 cup red onion, finely chopped
- 2 tbsp fresh basil, chopped
- Salt and pepper to taste

Instructions:

1. Heat olive oil in a pan over medium heat.
2. Add red onion and sauté until softened.

3. Add crumbled tofu, cherry tomatoes, and olives. Cook until tofu is lightly browned.

4. Season with salt and pepper, garnish with fresh basil.

5. Serve hot.

Nutrition Information:

- Calories: 250
- Protein: 15g
- Carbohydrates: 10g
- Fat: 18g
- Fiber: 4g
- Sugar: 2g
- Portion Size: 1 serving

Spinach and Feta Omelette

Ingredients:

- 3 eggs, beaten
- 1/2 cup fresh spinach, chopped
- 1/4 cup feta cheese, crumbled
- 1 tbsp olive oil
- Salt and pepper to taste

Instructions:

1. Heat olive oil in a pan over medium heat.
2. Pour beaten eggs into the pan.
3. Add spinach and feta on one half of the omelette.
4. Fold the omelette in half and cook until eggs are set.
5. Season with salt and pepper.
6. Serve warm.

Nutrition Information:

- Calories: 280
- Protein: 18g
- Carbohydrates: 3g
- Fat: 21g
- Fiber: 1g
- Sugar: 0g
- Portion Size: 1 serving

Quinoa Breakfast Bowl

Ingredients:

- 1/2 cup cooked quinoa
- 1/4 cup almonds, chopped
- 1/2 cup mixed berries (blueberries, strawberries)

- 1 tbsp honey
- 1/4 cup Greek yogurt

Instructions:

1. In a bowl, layer cooked quinoa.
2. Top with chopped almonds and mixed berries.
3. Drizzle honey over the mixture.
4. Add a dollop of Greek yogurt.
5. Mix before eating.

Nutrition Information:

- Calories: 320
- Protein: 12g
- Carbohydrates: 40g
- Fat: 14g
- Fiber: 6g
- Sugar: 12g
- Portion Size: 1 serving

Greek Yogurt Parfait

Ingredients:

- 1 cup Greek yogurt

- 1/4 cup granola
- 1/2 cup mixed berries (raspberries, blackberries)
- 1 tbsp honey
- 1 tbsp chia seeds

Instructions:

1. In a glass, layer Greek yogurt.
2. Add granola and mixed berries.
3. Drizzle honey over the layers.
4. Sprinkle chia seeds on top.
5. Repeat layers.
6. Enjoy this parfait!

Nutrition Information:

- Calories: 280
- Protein: 15g
- Carbohydrates: 35g
- Fat: 9g
- Fiber: 7g
- Sugar: 18g
- Portion Size: 1 serving

Avocado Toast with Cherry Tomatoes

Ingredients:

- 1 slice whole-grain bread
- 1/2 avocado, mashed
- 1/2 cup cherry tomatoes, sliced
- 1 tbsp lemon juice
- Salt and pepper to taste

Instructions:

1. Toast the whole-grain bread to your liking.
2. Spread mashed avocado on the toast.
3. Top with sliced cherry tomatoes.
4. Drizzle lemon juice over the top.
5. Season with salt and pepper.
6. Enjoy this nutrient-packed toast!

Nutrition Information:

- Calories: 220
- Protein: 5g
- Carbohydrates: 25g
- Fat: 13g

- Fiber: 8g
- Sugar: 2g
- Portion Size: 1 serving

Chickpea Flour Pancakes

Ingredients:
- 1 cup chickpea flour
- 1/2 cup almond milk
- 1/2 tsp baking powder
- 1/4 cup cherry tomatoes, diced
- 1/4 cup red bell pepper, chopped
- 1/4 cup fresh parsley, chopped

Instructions:
1. In a bowl, mix chickpea flour, almond milk, and baking powder.
2. Add diced cherry tomatoes, chopped red bell pepper, and fresh parsley.
3. Heat a pan and pour the batter to make pancakes.
4. Cook until edges are golden, then flip.
5. Serve warm.

Nutrition Information:

- Calories: 280
- Protein: 15g
- Carbohydrates: 30g
- Fat: 10g
- Fiber: 8g
- Sugar: 4g
- Portion Size: 1 serving

Mediterranean Veggie Frittata

Ingredients:

- 4 eggs, beaten
- 1/2 cup cherry tomatoes, halved
- 1/4 cup black olives, sliced
- 1/4 cup red onion, diced
- 1/2 cup spinach, chopped
- 1/4 cup feta cheese, crumbled
- Salt and pepper to taste

Instructions:

1. Preheat the oven to 375°F (190°C).

2. In an oven-safe pan, sauté cherry tomatoes, black olives, and red onion until softened.

3. Add chopped spinach and cook until wilted.

4. Pour beaten eggs over the veggies, sprinkle feta on top.

5. Season with salt and pepper.

6. Transfer the pan to the oven and bake until eggs are set.

7. Slice and serve.

Nutrition Information:

- Calories: 280
- Protein: 16g
- Carbohydrates: 10g
- Fat: 20g
- Fiber: 3g
- Sugar: 4g
- Portion Size: 1 serving

Almond and Berry Smoothie Bowl

Ingredients:

- 1/2 cup almond milk

- 1/2 banana, frozen
- 1/2 cup mixed berries (strawberries, blueberries)
- 2 tbsp almond butter
- 1 tbsp chia seeds
- 1/4 cup almonds, sliced

Instructions:

1. Blend almond milk, frozen banana, mixed berries, and almond butter until smooth.
2. Pour the smoothie into a bowl.
3. Top with chia seeds and sliced almonds.
4. Enjoy this refreshing and nutritious smoothie bowl.

Nutrition Information:

- Calories: 320
- Protein: 10g
- Carbohydrates: 30g
- Fat: 20g
- Fiber: 8g
- Sugar: 12g
- Portion Size: 1 serving

Zucchini and Tomato Breakfast Casserole

Ingredients:

- 2 zucchinis, thinly sliced
- 1 cup cherry tomatoes, halved
- 1/2 cup feta cheese, crumbled
- 4 eggs, beaten
- 1/4 cup fresh basil, chopped
- Salt and pepper to taste

Instructions:

1. Preheat the oven to 375°F (190°C).
2. In a greased baking dish, layer zucchini slices and cherry tomatoes.
3. Sprinkle crumbled feta over the vegetables.
4. In a bowl, beat eggs, add chopped basil, salt, and pepper.
5. Pour the egg mixture over the vegetables.
6. Bake until the eggs are set and the top is golden.
7. Slice and serve warm.

Nutrition Information:

- Calories: 260
- Protein: 15g
- Carbohydrates: 10g
- Fat: 18g
- Fiber: 3g
- Sugar: 5g
- Portion Size: 1 serving

Chia Seed Pudding with Berries

Ingredients:

- 1/4 cup chia seeds
- 1 cup almond milk
- 1/2 tsp vanilla extract
- 1 tbsp honey
- 1/2 cup mixed berries (raspberries, blackberries)

Instructions:

1. In a jar, mix chia seeds, almond milk, vanilla extract, and honey.
2. Stir well and refrigerate overnight.
3. In the morning, top with mixed berries.

4. Stir before enjoying this delightful chia seed pudding.

Nutrition Information:

- Calories: 220
- Protein: 6g
- Carbohydrates: 25g
- Fat: 12g
- Fiber: 10g
- Sugar: 8g
- Portion Size: 1 serving

Whole Grain Muesli with Nuts and Dried Fruits

Ingredients:

- 1/2 cup whole grain muesli
- 1/4 cup almonds, chopped
- 1/4 cup dried fruits (apricots, figs), chopped
- 1 cup Greek yogurt
- 1 tbsp honey

Instructions:

1. In a bowl, combine whole grain muesli, chopped almonds, and dried fruits.

2. Mix in Greek yogurt.

3. Drizzle honey over the top.

4. Stir well and let it sit for a few minutes.

5. Enjoy this wholesome and satisfying muesli.

Nutrition Information:

- Calories: 290
- Protein: 15g
- Carbohydrates: 30g
- Fat: 12g
- Fiber: 6g
- Sugar: 12g
- Portion Size: 1 serving

Eggplant and Mozzarella Breakfast Sandwich

Ingredients:

- 1 whole-grain English muffin

- 1/2 cup grilled eggplant slices
- 1/4 cup mozzarella cheese, sliced
- 1 egg, fried
- Salt and pepper to taste

Instructions:

1. Toast the whole-grain English muffin.
2. Layer grilled eggplant slices and mozzarella on one half.
3. Fry the egg and place it on top.
4. Season with salt and pepper.
5. Top with the other half of the muffin.
6. Indulge in this flavorful breakfast sandwich.

Nutrition Information:

- Calories: 320
- Protein: 16g
- Carbohydrates: 30g
- Fat: 15g
- Fiber: 6g
- Sugar: 4g
- Portion Size: 1 serving

Bulgur Porridge with Pistachios

Ingredients:

- 1/2 cup coarse bulgur
- 1 cup almond milk
- 1/4 cup pistachios, chopped
- 1 tbsp honey
- 1/2 tsp cinnamon

Instructions:

1. In a saucepan, combine bulgur and almond milk.
2. Bring to a simmer and cook until bulgur is tender.
3. Stir in chopped pistachios, honey, and cinnamon.
4. Cook for an additional few minutes.
5. Remove from heat and let it cool slightly before serving.

Nutrition Information:

- Calories: 270
- Protein: 8g
- Carbohydrates: 40g
- Fat: 10g
- Fiber: 8g

- Sugar: 8g
- Portion Size: 1 serving

Sweet Potato and Black Bean Hash

Ingredients:

- 1 sweet potato, diced
- 1/2 cup black beans, cooked
- 1/4 cup red bell pepper, diced
- 1/4 cup red onion, chopped
- 1 tbsp olive oil
- 1/2 tsp smoked paprika
- Salt and pepper to taste

Instructions:

1. In a skillet, heat olive oil over medium heat.
2. Add diced sweet potato, black beans, red bell pepper, and red onion.
3. Season with smoked paprika, salt, and pepper.
4. Cook until sweet potatoes are tender.
5. Serve hot as a delicious and hearty breakfast hash.

Nutrition Information:

- Calories: 290
- Protein: 9g
- Carbohydrates: 40g
- Fat: 10g
- Fiber: 10g
- Sugar: 8g
- Portion Size: 1 serving

Mediterranean-style Shakshuka

Ingredients:

- 2 tbsp olive oil
- 1/2 cup red bell pepper, diced
- 1/2 cup yellow bell pepper, diced
- 1/4 cup red onion, finely chopped
- 2 cloves garlic, minced
- 1 can (14 oz) diced tomatoes
- 1 tsp cumin
- 1 tsp paprika
- 1/2 tsp cayenne pepper (adjust to taste)
- Salt and pepper to taste
- 4 eggs

- Fresh parsley, chopped, for garnish

Instructions:

1. In a skillet, heat olive oil over medium heat.
2. Add red and yellow bell peppers, red onion, and garlic. Sauté until softened.
3. Pour in diced tomatoes and their juices.
4. Stir in cumin, paprika, cayenne pepper, salt, and pepper.
5. Simmer for 10-15 minutes until the sauce thickens.
6. Create small wells in the sauce and crack eggs into them.
7. Cover and cook until the eggs are set to your liking.
8. Garnish with fresh parsley and serve hot.

Nutrition Information:

- Calories: 280
- Protein: 14g
- Carbohydrates: 20g
- Fat: 16g
- Fiber: 5g
- Sugar: 10g
- Portion Size: 1 serving

Chapter 3: Lunch Recipes

These Mediterranean-inspired dishes are not just a treat for your taste buds but also cater to those managing Type 1 Diabetes. Each recipe is crafted to bring together the vibrant flavors of the region with a vegetarian twist.

Lentil and Vegetable Salad

Ingredients:

- 1 cup cooked lentils
- 1 cup cherry tomatoes, halved
- 1 cucumber, diced
- 1 bell pepper, chopped
- 1/4 cup red onion, finely sliced
- 2 tablespoons olive oil
- 1 tablespoon balsamic vinegar
- Salt and pepper to taste

Instructions:

1. In a large bowl, combine lentils, cherry tomatoes, cucumber, bell pepper, and red onion.

2. In a small bowl, whisk together olive oil, balsamic vinegar, salt, and pepper.

3. Pour the dressing over the salad and toss gently to combine.

4. Serve chilled.

Nutrition Information:

- Calories: 250
- Protein: 12g
- Carbohydrates: 35g
- Fat: 8g
- Fiber: 10g
- Sugar: 5g
- Portion Size: 1 serving

Greek Salad Wrap

Ingredients:

- 1 whole wheat wrap
- 1 cup mixed greens
- 1/2 cup cherry tomatoes, halved
- 1/4 cup cucumber, diced
- 2 tablespoons feta cheese, crumbled

- 1 tablespoon Kalamata olives, sliced
- 1 tablespoon Greek dressing

Instructions:

1. Lay out the whole wheat wrap and add mixed greens, cherry tomatoes, cucumber, feta cheese, and Kalamata olives.
2. Drizzle the Greek dressing over the ingredients.
3. Wrap tightly and secure with a toothpick if needed.
4. Slice in half and serve.

Nutrition Information:

- Calories: 300
- Protein: 10g
- Carbohydrates: 40g
- Fat: 12g
- Fiber: 8g
- Sugar: 5g
- Portion Size: 1 wrap

Mediterranean Quinoa Bowl

Ingredients:

- 1 cup cooked quinoa
- 1/2 cup cherry tomatoes, halved
- 1/4 cup red bell pepper, diced
- 1/4 cup cucumber, diced
- 2 tablespoons feta cheese, crumbled
- 1 tablespoon Kalamata olives, sliced
- 1 tablespoon olive oil
- 1 teaspoon lemon juice
- Salt and pepper to taste

Instructions:

1. In a bowl, combine quinoa, cherry tomatoes, red bell pepper, cucumber, feta cheese, and Kalamata olives.
2. Drizzle olive oil and lemon juice over the ingredients.
3. Season with salt and pepper, then toss gently to mix.
4. Serve at room temperature.

Nutrition Information:

- Calories: 280

- Protein: 8g

- Carbohydrates: 35g

- Fat: 12g

- Fiber: 6g

- Sugar: 3g

- Portion Size: 1 serving

Stuffed Bell Peppers with Couscous

Ingredients:

- 2 large bell peppers, halved

- 1 cup cooked couscous

- 1/2 cup black beans, drained and rinsed

- 1/4 cup corn kernels

- 1/4 cup red onion, finely chopped

- 1/2 cup tomato sauce

- 1 teaspoon cumin

- 1/2 teaspoon smoked paprika

- Salt and pepper to taste

Instructions:

1. Preheat the oven to 375°F (190°C).

2. In a bowl, mix cooked couscous, black beans, corn, red onion, tomato sauce, cumin, smoked paprika, salt, and pepper.
3. Stuff the bell peppers with the couscous mixture.
4. Bake for 25-30 minutes until peppers are tender.
5. Serve warm.

Nutrition Information:

- Calories: 320
- Protein: 10g
- Carbohydrates: 50g
- Fat: 5g
- Fiber: 8g
- Sugar: 5g
- Portion Size: 1 serving

Caprese Salad with Balsamic Glaze

Ingredients:

- 1 cup cherry tomatoes, halved
- 1 cup fresh mozzarella, cubed
- 1/4 cup fresh basil leaves
- 1 tablespoon balsamic glaze

- 1 tablespoon olive oil

- Salt and pepper to taste

Instructions:

1. Arrange cherry tomatoes, fresh mozzarella, and basil on a serving plate.
2. Drizzle with olive oil and balsamic glaze.
3. Season with salt and pepper.
4. Serve as a refreshing Caprese salad.

Nutrition Information:

- Calories: 280

- Protein: 14g

- Carbohydrates: 5g

- Fat: 22g

- Fiber: 1g

- Sugar: 2g

- Portion Size: 1 serving

Chickpea and Spinach Stew

Ingredients:

- 1 can (15 oz) chickpeas, drained and rinsed

- 2 cups fresh spinach
- 1 onion, finely chopped
- 2 cloves garlic, minced
- 1 can (14 oz) diced tomatoes
- 1 teaspoon cumin
- 1/2 teaspoon smoked paprika
- 1/4 teaspoon cayenne pepper
- Salt and pepper to taste

Instructions:

1. In a large pot, sauté onion and garlic until softened.
2. Add chickpeas, spinach, diced tomatoes, cumin, smoked paprika, cayenne pepper, salt, and pepper.
3. Simmer for 15-20 minutes.
4. Adjust seasoning as needed.
5. Serve hot.

Nutrition Information:

- Calories: 280
- Protein: 12g
- Carbohydrates: 45g
- Fat: 6g

- Fiber: 12g
- Sugar: 8g
- Portion Size: 1 serving

Roasted Vegetable and Hummus Wrap

Ingredients:

- 1 whole wheat wrap
- 1/2 cup hummus
- 1 cup mixed roasted vegetables (zucchini, bell peppers, eggplant)
- 1/4 cup baby spinach
- Salt and pepper to taste

Instructions:

1. Spread hummus on the whole wheat wrap.
2. Layer with mixed roasted vegetables and baby spinach.
3. Season with salt and pepper.
4. Roll tightly and slice in half.
5. Enjoy a nutritious wrap.

Nutrition Information:

- Calories: 320
- Protein: 10g
- Carbohydrates: 40g
- Fat: 14g
- Fiber: 8g
- Sugar: 5g
- Portion Size: 1 wrap

Tomato and Basil Bruschetta

Ingredients:

- 4 slices whole grain bread
- 2 cups cherry tomatoes, diced
- 1/4 cup fresh basil, chopped
- 2 cloves garlic, minced
- 2 tablespoons balsamic vinegar
- 1 tablespoon olive oil
- Salt and pepper to taste

Instructions:

1. Toast the whole grain bread slices.

2. In a bowl, combine diced cherry tomatoes, fresh basil, garlic, balsamic vinegar, olive oil, salt, and pepper.

3. Spoon the tomato mixture over the toasted bread.

4. Serve as a flavorful bruschetta.

Nutrition Information:

- Calories: 220
- Protein: 6g
- Carbohydrates: 30g
- Fat: 10g
- Fiber: 5g
- Sugar: 5g
- Portion Size: 1 serving

Mediterranean Chickpea Salad

Ingredients:

- 1 can (15 oz) chickpeas, drained and rinsed
- 1 cup cherry tomatoes, halved
- 1 cucumber, diced
- 1/4 cup red onion, finely chopped
- 1/4 cup feta cheese, crumbled

- 2 tablespoons black olives, sliced
- 2 tablespoons olive oil
- 1 tablespoon red wine vinegar
- Salt and pepper to taste

Instructions:

1. In a bowl, combine chickpeas, cherry tomatoes, cucumber, red onion, feta cheese, and black olives.
2. Drizzle olive oil and red wine vinegar over the ingredients.
3. Season with salt and pepper, then toss gently to combine.
4. Serve chilled.

Nutrition Information:

- Calories: 280
- Protein: 10g
- Carbohydrates: 35g
- Fat: 14g
- Fiber: 8g
- Sugar: 5g
- Portion Size: 1 serving

Eggplant and Mozzarella Panini

Ingredients:

- 1 whole grain ciabatta roll
- 1/2 cup grilled eggplant slices
- 2 slices fresh mozzarella
- 1 tablespoon pesto sauce
- 1 teaspoon olive oil

Instructions:

1. Slice the ciabatta roll in half.
2. Layer grilled eggplant, fresh mozzarella, and pesto sauce.
3. Close the sandwich and brush the outside with olive oil.
4. Grill until the cheese melts and the bread is crispy.
5. Slice and serve.

Nutrition Information:

- Calories: 350
- Protein: 12g
- Carbohydrates: 40g
- Fat: 18g

- Fiber: 6g
- Sugar: 4g
- Portion Size: 1 panini

Spinach and Feta Stuffed Mushrooms

Ingredients:

- 8 large mushrooms, stems removed
- 2 cups fresh spinach, chopped
- 1/2 cup feta cheese, crumbled
- 2 cloves garlic, minced
- 1 tablespoon olive oil
- Salt and pepper to taste

Instructions:

1. Preheat the oven to 375°F (190°C).
2. In a pan, sauté spinach and garlic in olive oil until wilted.
3. Mix the sautéed spinach with feta cheese.
4. Stuff each mushroom cap with the spinach and feta mixture.

5. Bake for 15-20 minutes.

6. Serve warm.

Nutrition Information:

- Calories: 180

- Protein: 8g

- Carbohydrates: 10g

- Fat: 14g

- Fiber: 3g

- Sugar: 2g

- Portion Size: 2 stuffed mushrooms

Cucumber and Avocado Sushi Rolls

Ingredients:

- 1 cup sushi rice, cooked

- 4 nori seaweed sheets

- 1 cucumber, julienned

- 1 avocado, sliced

- Soy sauce and wasabi for dipping

Instructions:

1. Place a nori sheet on a bamboo sushi mat.

2. Spread a thin layer of sushi rice over the nori.

3. Arrange cucumber and avocado slices along one edge.

4. Roll tightly using the sushi mat.

5. Slice into bite-sized pieces.

6. Serve with soy sauce and wasabi.

Nutrition Information:

- Calories: 220

- Protein: 5g

- Carbohydrates: 40g

- Fat: 6g

- Fiber: 5g

- Sugar: 2g

- Portion Size: 1 serving

Farro and Roasted Vegetable Bowl

Ingredients:

- 1 cup cooked farro

- 1 cup mixed roasted vegetables (carrots, bell peppers, zucchini)

- 1/4 cup crumbled goat cheese

- 2 tablespoons balsamic vinaigrette
- Fresh herbs for garnish

Instructions:

1. In a bowl, combine cooked farro and mixed roasted vegetables.
2. Top with crumbled goat cheese.
3. Drizzle with balsamic vinaigrette.
4. Garnish with fresh herbs.
5. Toss gently and serve.

Nutrition Information:

- Calories: 300
- Protein: 10g
- Carbohydrates: 45g
- Fat: 8g
- Fiber: 10g
- Sugar: 5g
- Portion Size: 1 serving

Mediterranean Pita Sandwich

Ingredients:

- 2 whole wheat pita pockets
- 1/2 cup hummus
- 1/2 cup cherry tomatoes, halved
- 1/4 cup cucumber, sliced
- 1/4 cup red onion, thinly sliced
- 1/4 cup feta cheese, crumbled
- Fresh mint leaves for garnish

Instructions:

1. Cut the pita pockets in half to form pockets.
2. Spread hummus inside each pocket.
3. Fill with cherry tomatoes, cucumber, red onion, and feta cheese.
4. Garnish with fresh mint leaves.
5. Serve as a refreshing pita sandwich.

Nutrition Information:

- Calories: 280
- Protein: 9g
- Carbohydrates: 40g

- Fat: 10g
- Fiber: 8g
- Sugar: 5g
- Portion Size: 1 sandwich

Cauliflower and Chickpea Curry

Ingredients:

- 1 tablespoon coconut oil
- 1 onion, chopped
- 2 cloves garlic, minced
- 1 tablespoon curry powder
- 1 teaspoon cumin
- 1 teaspoon turmeric
- 1 can (15 oz) chickpeas, drained and rinsed
- 1 small cauliflower, cut into florets
- 1 can (14 oz) diced tomatoes
- 1 cup coconut milk
- Salt and pepper to taste
- Fresh cilantro for garnish

Instructions:

1. In a large pot, sauté onion and garlic in coconut oil until softened.
2. Add curry powder, cumin, and turmeric, stirring to combine.
3. Add chickpeas, cauliflower, diced tomatoes, and coconut milk.
4. Simmer until cauliflower is tender.
5. Season with salt and pepper.
6. Garnish with fresh cilantro and serve.

Nutrition Information:

- Calories: 320
- Protein: 10g
- Carbohydrates: 45g
- Fat: 15g
- Fiber: 12g
- Sugar: 8g
- Portion Size: 1 serving

Chapter 4: Dinner Recipes

These dinner recipes promise to tantalize your taste buds while maintaining a healthy balance for those managing Type 1 Diabetes. Each dish is crafted with a symphony of fresh ingredients and vibrant flavors, embodying the essence of the Mediterranean diet.

Mediterranean Stuffed Zucchini Boats

Ingredients:

- Zucchini (4 medium)
- Cherry tomatoes (1 cup, halved)
- Quinoa (1 cup, cooked)
- Feta cheese (1/2 cup, crumbled)
- Kalamata olives (1/4 cup, chopped)
- Fresh basil (2 tablespoons, chopped)
- Olive oil (2 tablespoons)
- Salt and pepper to taste

Instructions:

1. Preheat the oven to 375°F (190°C).

2. Cut zucchinis in half lengthwise, scoop out the seeds to create boats.

3. In a bowl, mix cooked quinoa, cherry tomatoes, feta, olives, and basil.

4. Stuff the zucchini boats with the mixture.

5. Drizzle with olive oil, sprinkle with salt and pepper.

6. Bake for 25-30 minutes or until zucchinis are tender.

7. Serve warm.

Nutrition Information:

- Calories: 210
- Protein: 8g
- Carbohydrates: 25g
- Fat: 10g
- Fiber: 5g
- Sugar: 4g
- Portion Size: 2 boats

Baked Eggplant Parmesan

Ingredients:

- Eggplant (1 large, sliced)
- Tomato sauce (2 cups)
- Mozzarella cheese (1 cup, shredded)
- Parmesan cheese (1/2 cup, grated)
- Bread crumbs (1/2 cup)
- Fresh basil (1/4 cup, chopped)
- Olive oil (2 tablespoons)
- Salt and pepper to taste

Instructions:

1. Preheat the oven to 375°F (190°C).
2. Dip eggplant slices in beaten egg, then coat with breadcrumbs.
3. Arrange eggplant slices in a baking dish, layer with tomato sauce, mozzarella, and Parmesan.
4. Repeat layers and top with fresh basil.
5. Drizzle with olive oil, season with salt and pepper.
6. Bake for 30-35 minutes until golden and bubbly.
7. Allow to cool slightly before serving.

Nutrition Information:

- Calories: 280
- Protein: 12g
- Carbohydrates: 20g
- Fat: 18g
- Fiber: 6g
- Sugar: 8g
- Portion Size: 1 cup

Lemon Garlic Orzo with Roasted Vegetables

Ingredients:

- Orzo pasta (1 cup, uncooked)
- Zucchini (1, diced)
- Bell peppers (2, diced)
- Cherry tomatoes (1 cup)
- Garlic (4 cloves, minced)
- Lemon juice (2 tablespoons)
- Olive oil (3 tablespoons)
- Fresh parsley (2 tablespoons, chopped)
- Salt and pepper to taste

Instructions:

1. Cook orzo according to package instructions.

2. In a bowl, toss zucchini, bell peppers, and cherry tomatoes with olive oil, garlic, salt, and pepper.

3. Roast vegetables in the oven at 400°F (200°C) for 20-25 minutes.

4. Mix cooked orzo with roasted vegetables, lemon juice, and fresh parsley.

5. Drizzle with extra olive oil if desired.

6. Serve warm.

Nutrition Information:

- Calories: 320
- Protein: 8g
- Carbohydrates: 45g
- Fat: 12g
- Fiber: 6g
- Sugar: 5g
- Portion Size: 1 cup

Artichoke and Sundried Tomato Risotto

Ingredients:

- Arborio rice (1 cup)
- Artichoke hearts (1 cup, chopped)
- Sundried tomatoes (1/2 cup, chopped)
- Vegetable broth (4 cups, heated)
- White wine (1/2 cup)
- Parmesan cheese (1/2 cup, grated)
- Onion (1, finely chopped)
- Garlic (2 cloves, minced)
- Olive oil (2 tablespoons)
- Fresh basil (1/4 cup, chopped)
- Salt and pepper to taste

Instructions:

1. In a pan, sauté onion and garlic in olive oil until translucent.
2. Add Arborio rice and stir until lightly toasted.
3. Pour in white wine and cook until mostly evaporated.
4. Begin adding warm vegetable broth, one ladle at a time, stirring until absorbed.

5. Continue until rice is creamy and al dente.

6. Stir in artichoke hearts, sundried tomatoes, Parmesan, and fresh basil.

7. Season with salt and pepper to taste.

8. Serve hot.

Nutrition Information:

- Calories: 350
- Protein: 10g
- Carbohydrates: 50g
- Fat: 12g
- Fiber: 4g
- Sugar: 3g
- Portion Size: 1 cup

Quinoa-Stuffed Bell Peppers

Ingredients:

- Bell peppers (4, halved and deseeded)
- Quinoa (1 cup, cooked)
- Black beans (1/2 cup, cooked)
- Corn kernels (1/2 cup)
- Salsa (1/2 cup)

- Cumin (1 teaspoon)
- Chili powder (1 teaspoon)
- Lime juice (2 tablespoons)
- Fresh cilantro (2 tablespoons, chopped)
- Avocado (1, sliced)
- Salt and pepper to taste

Instructions:

1. Preheat the oven to 375°F (190°C).
2. In a bowl, mix quinoa, black beans, corn, salsa, cumin, chili powder, lime juice, and cilantro.
3. Stuff bell peppers with the quinoa mixture.
4. Bake for 25-30 minutes until peppers are tender.
5. Top with avocado slices before serving.
6. Garnish with additional cilantro if desired.

Nutrition Information:

- Calories: 280
- Protein: 9g
- Carbohydrates: 45g
- Fat: 8g
- Fiber: 10g

- Sugar: 5g
- Portion Size: 2 halves

Spaghetti Aglio e Olio with Cherry Tomatoes

Ingredients:

- Whole wheat spaghetti (8 oz, cooked)
- Cherry tomatoes (1 cup, halved)
- Garlic (4 cloves, thinly sliced)
- Red pepper flakes (1/2 teaspoon)
- Fresh parsley (1/4 cup, chopped)
- Olive oil (3 tablespoons)
- Grated Parmesan cheese (1/4 cup)
- Salt and pepper to taste

Instructions:

1. Cook spaghetti according to package instructions.
2. In a pan, sauté garlic and red pepper flakes in olive oil until garlic is golden.
3. Add cherry tomatoes and cook until softened.

4. Toss cooked spaghetti in the tomato and garlic mixture.

5. Season with salt and pepper, top with fresh parsley and Parmesan.

6. Serve immediately.

Nutrition Information:

- Calories: 340
- Protein: 10g
- Carbohydrates: 45g
- Fat: 12g
- Fiber: 6g
- Sugar: 3g
- Portion Size: 1 cup

Sweet Potato and Chickpea Tagine

Ingredients:

- Sweet potatoes (2, peeled and diced)
- Chickpeas (1 can, drained and rinsed)
- Onion (1, finely chopped)
- Garlic (3 cloves, minced)
- Vegetable broth (1 cup)

- Canned tomatoes (1 can, diced)
- Ground cumin (1 teaspoon)
- Ground coriander (1 teaspoon)
- Cinnamon (1/2 teaspoon)
- Turmeric (1/2 teaspoon)
- Fresh cilantro (1/4 cup, chopped)
- Olive oil (2 tablespoons)
- Salt and pepper to taste

Instructions:

1. In a large pot, sauté onion and garlic in olive oil until softened.
2. Add sweet potatoes, chickpeas, vegetable broth, diced tomatoes, cumin, coriander, cinnamon, and turmeric.
3. Bring to a simmer and cook until sweet potatoes are tender.
4. Season with salt and pepper.
5. Garnish with fresh cilantro before serving.
6. Serve over couscous or rice.

Nutrition Information:

- Calories: 320
- Protein: 10g
- Carbohydrates: 55g
- Fat: 8g
- Fiber: 12g
- Sugar: 8g
- Portion Size: 1 cup

Mediterranean Lentil Soup

Ingredients:

- Brown lentils (1 cup, dried)
- Carrots (2, diced)
- Celery (2 stalks, diced)
- Onion (1, finely chopped)
- Garlic (3 cloves, minced)
- Vegetable broth (6 cups)
- Canned tomatoes (1 can, crushed)
- Ground cumin (1 teaspoon)
- Smoked paprika (1 teaspoon)
- Bay leaves (2)
- Fresh parsley (1/4 cup, chopped)

- Olive oil (2 tablespoons)
- Salt and pepper to taste

Instructions:

1. Rinse lentils and set aside.
2. In a large pot, sauté onion and garlic in olive oil until translucent.
3. Add lentils, carrots, celery, vegetable broth, crushed tomatoes, cumin, paprika, and bay leaves.
4. Simmer until lentils are tender.
5. Season with salt and pepper, garnish with fresh parsley.
6. Discard bay leaves before serving.
7. Enjoy hot.

Nutrition Information:

- Calories: 280
- Protein: 14g
- Carbohydrates: 45g
- Fat: 6g
- Fiber: 12g
- Sugar: 8g

- Portion Size: 1 cup

Grilled Portobello Mushrooms with Polenta

Ingredients:

- Portobello mushrooms (4, cleaned and stems removed)
- Polenta (1 cup, sliced)
- Balsamic vinegar (2 tablespoons)
- Olive oil (3 tablespoons)
- Garlic (2 cloves, minced)
- Fresh thyme (1 tablespoon, chopped)
- Salt and pepper to taste

Instructions:

1. Preheat the grill or grill pan.
2. In a bowl, whisk together balsamic vinegar, olive oil, garlic, and thyme.
3. Brush the Portobello mushrooms with the mixture.
4. Grill mushrooms for 4-5 minutes per side.

5. Meanwhile, cook polenta according to package instructions.

6. Serve grilled mushrooms over a bed of polenta.

7. Season with salt and pepper.

Nutrition Information:

- Calories: 290
- Protein: 8g
- Carbohydrates: 35g
- Fat: 14g
- Fiber: 6g
- Sugar: 2g
- Portion Size: 1 mushroom and 1/2 cup polenta

Ratatouille with Herbed Couscous

Ingredients:

- Eggplant (1, diced)
- Zucchini (2, diced)
- Bell peppers (2, diced)
- Onion (1, diced)
- Garlic (3 cloves, minced)
- Tomatoes (4, diced)

- Tomato paste (2 tablespoons)
- Olive oil (3 tablespoons)
- Herbed couscous (2 cups, cooked)
- Fresh thyme (1 tablespoon, chopped)
- Fresh basil (1/4 cup, chopped)
- Salt and pepper to taste

Instructions:

1. In a large pan, sauté onion and garlic in olive oil until softened.
2. Add eggplant, zucchini, bell peppers, tomatoes, and tomato paste.
3. Cook until vegetables are tender.
4. Season with salt, pepper, fresh thyme, and basil.
5. Serve over herbed couscous.

Nutrition Information:

- Calories: 310
- Protein: 10g
- Carbohydrates: 50g
- Fat: 8g
- Fiber: 10g

- Sugar: 8g
- Portion Size: 1 cup

Spinach and Feta Stuffed Chicken Breast

Ingredients:

- Chicken breasts (4, boneless and skinless)
- Spinach (2 cups, chopped)
- Feta cheese (1/2 cup, crumbled)
- Garlic (3 cloves, minced)
- Olive oil (2 tablespoons)
- Lemon juice (2 tablespoons)
- Dried oregano (1 teaspoon)
- Salt and pepper to taste

Instructions:

1. Preheat the oven to 375°F (190°C).
2. In a pan, sauté garlic in olive oil until fragrant.
3. Add chopped spinach and cook until wilted.
4. Remove from heat, stir in feta, lemon juice, oregano, salt, and pepper.

5. Cut a pocket into each chicken breast.

6. Stuff each pocket with the spinach and feta mixture.

7. Bake for 25-30 minutes or until chicken is cooked through.

8. Serve hot.

Nutrition Information:

- Calories: 280

- Protein: 35g

- Carbohydrates: 4g

- Fat: 12g

- Fiber: 2g

- Sugar: 1g

- Portion Size: 1 stuffed chicken breast

Pesto Pasta with Cherry Tomatoes

Ingredients:

- Whole wheat pasta (8 oz, cooked)

- Cherry tomatoes (1 cup, halved)

- Pesto sauce (1/2 cup)

- Pine nuts (1/4 cup, toasted)

- Parmesan cheese (1/4 cup, grated)

- Fresh basil (1/4 cup, chopped)
- Olive oil (2 tablespoons)
- Salt and pepper to taste

Instructions:

1. Cook pasta according to package instructions.
2. In a bowl, mix cooked pasta, cherry tomatoes, pesto sauce, pine nuts, Parmesan, and fresh basil.
3. Drizzle with olive oil, season with salt and pepper.
4. Toss until well combined.
5. Serve warm.

Nutrition Information:

- Calories: 350
- Protein: 10g
- Carbohydrates: 45g
- Fat: 15g
- Fiber: 8g
- Sugar: 3g
- Portion Size: 1 cup

Mediterranean Baked Cod

Ingredients:

- Cod fillets (4, about 6 oz each)
- Cherry tomatoes (1 cup, halved)
- Kalamata olives (1/2 cup, sliced)
- Red onion (1/2, thinly sliced)
- Garlic (3 cloves, minced)
- Olive oil (3 tablespoons)
- Lemon juice (2 tablespoons)
- Fresh oregano (1 tablespoon, chopped)
- Salt and pepper to taste

Instructions:

1. Preheat the oven to 400°F (200°C).
2. Place cod fillets in a baking dish.
3. In a bowl, mix cherry tomatoes, olives, red onion, garlic, olive oil, lemon juice, oregano, salt, and pepper.
4. Spoon the tomato mixture over the cod.
5. Bake for 15-20 minutes or until the cod is cooked through.
6. Serve hot.

Nutrition Information:

- Calories: 280
- Protein: 30g
- Carbohydrates: 8g
- Fat: 15g
- Fiber: 2g
- Sugar: 3g
- Portion Size: 1 fillet

Zoodles with Tomato and Basil Sauce

Ingredients:

- Zucchini (4, spiralized into zoodles)
- Tomatoes (4, diced)
- Garlic (3 cloves, minced)
- Fresh basil (1/2 cup, chopped)
- Olive oil (2 tablespoons)
- Balsamic vinegar (2 tablespoons)
- Red pepper flakes (1/2 teaspoon)
- Salt and pepper to taste

Instructions:

1. In a pan, sauté garlic in olive oil until fragrant.

2. Add diced tomatoes, balsamic vinegar, and red pepper flakes.

3. Cook until tomatoes break down into a sauce.

4. Add zoodles and toss until heated through.

5. Stir in fresh basil and season with salt and pepper.

6. Serve immediately.

Nutrition Information:

- Calories: 180

- Protein: 5g

- Carbohydrates: 15g

- Fat: 10g

- Fiber: 5g

- Sugar: 8g

- Portion Size: 1 cup

Vegan Paella

Ingredients:

- Arborio rice (1 cup)

- Vegetable broth (4 cups, heated)

- Onion (1, finely chopped)
- Bell peppers (2, diced)
- Tomatoes (2, diced)
- Green beans (1 cup, chopped)
- Artichoke hearts (1 cup, quartered)
- Smoked paprika (1 teaspoon)
- Saffron threads (1/4 teaspoon, dissolved in hot water)
- Olive oil (2 tablespoons)
- Lemon wedges for serving
- Salt and pepper to taste

Instructions:

1. In a paella pan, sauté onion in olive oil until translucent.
2. Add bell peppers, tomatoes, green beans, and artichoke hearts.
3. Stir in rice, smoked paprika, saffron mixture, and season with salt and pepper.
4. Pour in heated vegetable broth and bring to a simmer.
5. Cook until rice is tender and liquid is absorbed.
6. Garnish with lemon wedges before serving.

7. Serve hot.

Nutrition Information:

- Calories: 320
- Protein: 6g
- Carbohydrates: 65g
- Fat: 5g
- Fiber: 8g
- Sugar: 5g
- Portion Size: 1 cup

Chapter 5: Snacks and Appetizers

These mouthwatering bites are not only a treat for your taste buds but are also thoughtfully designed to fit into a Mediterranean diet, offering a perfect blend of flavors and nutrition.

Hummus with Veggie Sticks

Ingredients:

- 1 can (15 oz) chickpeas, drained and rinsed
- 3 tbsp tahini
- 3 tbsp olive oil
- 2 cloves garlic, minced
- 1 tsp cumin
- Salt and pepper to taste
- Assorted vegetable sticks (carrots, cucumber, bell peppers) for dipping

Instructions:

1. In a food processor, combine chickpeas, tahini, olive oil, garlic, cumin, salt, and pepper.

2. Blend until smooth and creamy.

3. Serve with a variety of fresh vegetable sticks.

Nutrition Information:

- Calories: 120 per serving

- Protein: 4g

- Carbohydrates: 14g

- Fat: 6g

- Fiber: 3g

- Sugar: 1g

- Portion Size: 2 tbsp hummus with veggie sticks

Mediterranean Bruschetta

Ingredients:

- 4 ripe tomatoes, diced

- 1/4 cup red onion, finely chopped

- 2 cloves garlic, minced

- 1/4 cup fresh basil, chopped

- 2 tbsp extra virgin olive oil

- Salt and pepper to taste

- Baguette slices for serving

Instructions:

1. In a bowl, combine tomatoes, red onion, garlic, basil, olive oil, salt, and pepper.

2. Spoon the mixture onto baguette slices.

Nutrition Information:

- Calories: 80 per serving
- Protein: 2g
- Carbohydrates: 12g
- Fat: 3g
- Fiber: 2g
- Sugar: 3g
- Portion Size: 2 bruschetta slices

Olive and Artichoke Tapenade

Ingredients:

- 1 cup Kalamata olives, pitted
- 1 cup marinated artichoke hearts
- 2 tbsp capers
- 2 tbsp fresh parsley, chopped
- 1 clove garlic, minced
- 3 tbsp extra virgin olive oil

- Crackers or whole-grain bread for serving

Instructions:

1. In a food processor, pulse olives, artichoke hearts, capers, parsley, garlic, and olive oil until coarsely chopped.
2. Spread on crackers or whole-grain bread.

Nutrition Information:

- Calories: 90 per serving
- Protein: 1g
- Carbohydrates: 4g
- Fat: 8g
- Fiber: 2g
- Sugar: 0g
- Portion Size: 2 tbsp tapenade with crackers

Greek Yogurt Dip with Cucumber

Ingredients:

- 1 cup Greek yogurt
- 1/2 cucumber, finely diced
- 1 tbsp fresh dill, chopped

- 1 tbsp lemon juice

- Salt and pepper to taste

- Pita chips for dipping

Instructions:

1. In a bowl, combine Greek yogurt, cucumber, dill, lemon juice, salt, and pepper.

2. Stir until well mixed.

3. Serve with pita chips.

Nutrition Information:

- Calories: 60 per serving

- Protein: 3g

- Carbohydrates: 5g

- Fat: 3g

- Fiber: 0g

- Sugar: 3g

- Portion Size: 3 tbsp dip with pita chips

Roasted Red Pepper and Feta Dip

Ingredients:

- 2 large red bell peppers, roasted and peeled

- 1/2 cup feta cheese, crumbled
- 2 tbsp Greek yogurt
- 1 clove garlic, minced
- 1 tbsp olive oil
- 1/2 tsp red pepper flakes (optional)
- Pita bread wedges for dipping

Instructions:

1. In a blender, combine roasted red peppers, feta cheese, Greek yogurt, garlic, olive oil, and red pepper flakes.
2. Blend until smooth.
3. Serve with pita bread wedges.

Nutrition Information:

- Calories: 100 per serving
- Protein: 4g
- Carbohydrates: 6g
- Fat: 7g
- Fiber: 1g
- Sugar: 3g
- Portion Size: 2 tbsp dip with pita wedges

Stuffed Grape Leaves with Tzatziki

Ingredients:

- 1 cup grape leaves, blanched
- 1/2 cup cooked quinoa
- 1/4 cup pine nuts, toasted
- 2 tbsp fresh mint, chopped
- 2 tbsp lemon juice
- Tzatziki sauce for dipping

Instructions:

1. In a bowl, mix cooked quinoa, pine nuts, mint, and lemon juice.
2. Spoon the mixture onto grape leaves and roll them up.
3. Serve with tzatziki sauce.

Nutrition Information:

- Calories: 120 per serving
- Protein: 3g
- Carbohydrates: 10g
- Fat: 8g
- Fiber: 2g

- Sugar: 1g
- Portion Size: 3 stuffed grape leaves with tzatziki

Spicy Chickpea Roast

Ingredients:

- 2 cans (15 oz each) chickpeas, drained and rinsed
- 2 tbsp olive oil
- 1 tsp smoked paprika
- 1/2 tsp cayenne pepper
- 1 tsp cumin
- Salt and pepper to taste

Instructions:

1. Preheat the oven to 400°F (200°C).
2. In a bowl, toss chickpeas with olive oil, smoked paprika, cayenne pepper, cumin, salt, and pepper.
3. Spread evenly on a baking sheet and roast for 20-25 minutes until crispy.
4. Allow to cool before serving.

Nutrition Information:

- Calories: 150 per serving

- Protein: 6g

- Carbohydrates: 22g

- Fat: 5g

- Fiber: 6g

- Sugar: 3g

- Portion Size: 1/2 cup spicy chickpeas

Sundried Tomato and White Bean Dip

Ingredients:

- 1 can (15 oz) cannellini beans, drained and rinsed

- 1/4 cup sundried tomatoes, soaked in hot water and drained

- 2 cloves garlic, minced

- 2 tbsp lemon juice

- 3 tbsp olive oil

- Salt and pepper to taste

- Whole-grain crackers for dipping

Instructions:

1. In a food processor, blend cannellini beans, sundried tomatoes, garlic, lemon juice, olive oil, salt, and pepper until smooth.

2. Serve with whole-grain crackers.

Nutrition Information:

- Calories: 80 per serving
- Protein: 3g
- Carbohydrates: 11g
- Fat: 4g
- Fiber: 3g
- Sugar: 1g
- Portion Size: 2 tbsp dip with crackers

Greek Spanakopita Bites

Ingredients:

- 1 package phyllo dough, thawed
- 2 cups fresh spinach, chopped
- 1 cup feta cheese, crumbled
- 1/4 cup fresh dill, chopped
- 1/4 cup olive oil

- 1/4 cup pine nuts, toasted

Instructions:

1. Preheat the oven to 375°F (190°C).

2. In a bowl, mix spinach, feta, dill, and pine nuts.

3. Cut the phyllo dough into small squares and place a spoonful of the spinach mixture in the center.

4. Fold into bite-sized triangles and brush with olive oil.

5. Bake for 15-20 minutes or until golden brown.

Nutrition Information:

- Calories: 120 per serving

- Protein: 4g

- Carbohydrates: 12g

- Fat: 7g

- Fiber: 1g

- Sugar: 0g

- Portion Size: 3 spanakopita bites

Roasted Garlic and White Bean Hummus

Ingredients:

- 1 can (15 oz) white beans, drained and rinsed
- 1 head garlic, roasted
- 3 tbsp tahini
- 2 tbsp lemon juice
- 2 tbsp olive oil
- Salt and pepper to taste
- Whole-grain pita chips for dipping

Instructions:

1. In a food processor, blend white beans, roasted garlic, tahini, lemon juice, olive oil, salt, and pepper until smooth.
2. Serve with whole-grain pita chips.

Nutrition Information:

- Calories: 90 per serving
- Protein: 3g
- Carbohydrates: 12g
- Fat: 4g

- Fiber: 3g

- Sugar: 1g

- Portion Size: 2 tbsp hummus with pita chips

Mediterranean Stuffed Mushrooms

Ingredients:

- 12 large mushrooms, stems removed

- 1 cup spinach, chopped

- 1/2 cup feta cheese, crumbled

- 2 tbsp sun-dried tomatoes, chopped

- 1 clove garlic, minced

- 1 tbsp olive oil

- Salt and pepper to taste

Instructions:

1. Preheat the oven to 375°F (190°C).

2. In a skillet, sauté spinach, feta, sun-dried tomatoes, garlic, olive oil, salt, and pepper until spinach is wilted.

3. Stuff each mushroom cap with the mixture.

4. Bake for 15-20 minutes or until mushrooms are tender.

Nutrition Information:

- Calories: 70 per serving
- Protein: 4g
- Carbohydrates: 5g
- Fat: 5g
- Fiber: 2g
- Sugar: 2g
- Portion Size: 2 stuffed mushrooms

Pistachio and Cranberry Energy Bites

Ingredients:

- 1 cup rolled oats
- 1/2 cup pistachios, chopped
- 1/2 cup dried cranberries, chopped
- 1/3 cup honey
- 1/2 cup almond butter
- 1 tsp vanilla extract
- Shredded coconut for coating

Instructions:

1. In a bowl, combine rolled oats, pistachios, cranberries, honey, almond butter, and vanilla extract.
2. Roll into bite-sized balls and coat with shredded coconut.
3. Refrigerate for at least 30 minutes before serving.

Nutrition Information:

- Calories: 100 per serving
- Protein: 3g
- Carbohydrates: 12g
- Fat: 5g
- Fiber: 2g
- Sugar: 7g
- Portion Size: 2 energy bites

Baked Zucchini Fries

Ingredients:

- 2 large zucchinis, cut into fries
- 1 cup breadcrumbs
- 1/4 cup Parmesan cheese, grated

- 1 tsp dried oregano
- 1/2 tsp garlic powder
- Salt and pepper to taste
- Olive oil spray

Instructions:

1. Preheat the oven to 425°F (220°C).
2. In a bowl, mix breadcrumbs, Parmesan cheese, oregano, garlic powder, salt, and pepper.
3. Dip zucchini fries in the breadcrumb mixture, ensuring an even coating.
4. Place on a baking sheet, spray with olive oil, and bake for 20-25 minutes or until golden brown.

Nutrition Information:

- Calories: 80 per serving
- Protein: 3g
- Carbohydrates: 12g
- Fat: 2g
- Fiber: 2g
- Sugar: 3g
- Portion Size: 10 zucchini fries

Avocado and Tomato Salsa

Ingredients:

- 2 ripe avocados, diced
- 1 cup cherry tomatoes, quartered
- 1/4 cup red onion, finely chopped
- 1/4 cup fresh cilantro, chopped
- 1 lime, juiced
- Salt and pepper to taste
- Whole-grain tortilla chips for dipping

Instructions:

1. In a bowl, combine avocados, cherry tomatoes, red onion, cilantro, lime juice, salt, and pepper.
2. Mix gently and serve with whole-grain tortilla chips.

Nutrition Information:

- Calories: 90 per serving
- Protein: 2g
- Carbohydrates: 8g
- Fat: 6g
- Fiber: 4g
- Sugar: 2g

- Portion Size: 1/2 cup salsa with chips

Caprese Skewers

Ingredients:

- 1 pint cherry tomatoes
- 1 package fresh mozzarella balls
- Fresh basil leaves
- Balsamic glaze for drizzling
- Sea salt and black pepper to taste

Instructions:

1. Thread a cherry tomato, a mozzarella ball, and a fresh basil leaf onto small skewers.
2. Arrange the skewers on a serving platter.
3. Drizzle with balsamic glaze and sprinkle with sea salt and black pepper before serving.

Nutrition Information:

- Calories: 50 per serving
- Protein: 3g
- Carbohydrates: 2g
- Fat: 3g

- Fiber: 1g
- Sugar: 1g
- Portion Size: 2 skewers

Chapter 6: Desserts

These desserts not only satiate your sweet cravings but also align with the principles of the Mediterranean lifestyle. Let's explore a diverse array of desserts, each carefully crafted with wholesome ingredients to strike a perfect balance of taste and nutrition.

Greek Yogurt with Honey and Nuts

Ingredients:

- 1 cup Greek yogurt
- 1 tablespoon honey
- 2 tablespoons mixed nuts (almonds, walnuts, pistachios)

Instructions:

1. In a bowl, spoon out the Greek yogurt.
2. Drizzle honey evenly over the yogurt.
3. Sprinkle mixed nuts on top.
4. Gently mix and enjoy!

Nutrition Information (per serving):

- Calories: 250
- Protein: 15g
- Carbohydrates: 20g
- Fat: 12g
- Fiber: 2g
- Sugar: 15g
- Portion Size: 1 serving

Mixed Berry Sorbet

Ingredients:

- 2 cups mixed berries (strawberries, blueberries, raspberries)
- 1/4 cup honey
- 1 tablespoon lemon juice

Instructions:

1. Blend berries, honey, and lemon juice until smooth.
2. Pour the mixture into a shallow dish.
3. Freeze for 4 hours, stirring every hour.
4. Scoop and serve!

Nutrition Information (per serving):

- Calories: 120
- Protein: 1g
- Carbohydrates: 30g
- Fat: 0.5g
- Fiber: 5g
- Sugar: 22g
- Portion Size: 1/2 cup

Almond Flour Orange Cake

Ingredients:

- 1 1/2 cups almond flour
- 1/2 cup honey
- 3 eggs
- Zest of 1 orange
- 1/4 cup orange juice
- 1 teaspoon baking powder

Instructions:

1. Preheat oven to 350°F (175°C).
2. Mix almond flour, honey, eggs, orange zest, orange juice, and baking powder.

3. Pour into a cake pan and bake for 25-30 minutes.

4. Allow to cool before slicing.

Nutrition Information (per serving):

- Calories: 180

- Protein: 6g

- Carbohydrates: 15g

- Fat: 12g

- Fiber: 3g

- Sugar: 10g

- Portion Size: 1 slice

Chocolate-Dipped Strawberries

Ingredients:

- 12 fresh strawberries

- 1/2 cup dark chocolate, melted

Instructions:

1. Dip each strawberry into melted chocolate.

2. Place on a parchment-lined tray.

3. Chill in the fridge until the chocolate sets.

4. Enjoy the sweet combination!

Nutrition Information (per serving):

- Calories: 60
- Protein: 1g
- Carbohydrates: 10g
- Fat: 3g
- Fiber: 2g
- Sugar: 6g
- Portion Size: 3 strawberries

Pistachio and Fig Energy Bars

Ingredients:

- 1 cup dried figs, chopped
- 1 cup pistachios, shelled
- 1/2 cup rolled oats
- 1/4 cup honey
- 1/2 teaspoon vanilla extract

Instructions:

1. Blend figs, pistachios, oats, honey, and vanilla in a food processor.
2. Press the mixture into a lined pan.
3. Refrigerate for 2 hours, then cut into bars.

Nutrition Information (per serving):

- Calories: 180
- Protein: 4g
- Carbohydrates: 25g
- Fat: 8g
- Fiber: 5g
- Sugar: 15g
- Portion Size: 1 bar

Mediterranean Fruit Salad

Ingredients:

- 2 cups mixed fresh fruits (grapes, melon, oranges, berries)
- 1 tablespoon fresh mint, chopped
- 1 tablespoon balsamic glaze

Instructions:

1. Combine fresh fruits in a bowl.
2. Sprinkle chopped mint and drizzle balsamic glaze.
3. Toss gently and serve chilled.

Nutrition Information (per serving):

- Calories: 80

- Protein: 1g

- Carbohydrates: 20g

- Fat: 0.5g

- Fiber: 3g

- Sugar: 15g

- Portion Size: 1 cup

Olive Oil and Lemon Cake

Ingredients:

- 1 1/2 cups whole wheat flour

- 1/2 cup olive oil

- 1/2 cup honey

- 3 eggs

- Zest of 1 lemon

- 1/4 cup lemon juice

- 1 teaspoon baking powder

Instructions:

1. Preheat oven to 350°F (175°C).

2. Mix whole wheat flour, olive oil, honey, eggs, lemon zest, lemon juice, and baking powder.

3. Pour into a cake pan and bake for 30-35 minutes.

4. Let it cool before serving.

Nutrition Information (per serving):

- Calories: 200
- Protein: 5g
- Carbohydrates: 20g
- Fat: 12g
- Fiber: 2g
- Sugar: 10g
- Portion Size: 1 slice

Date and Nut Balls

Ingredients:

- 1 cup dates, pitted
- 1 cup mixed nuts (almonds, walnuts)
- 1/2 cup shredded coconut
- 1 tablespoon chia seeds

Instructions:

1. Blend dates and mixed nuts in a food processor.
2. Add shredded coconut and chia seeds, blend until a sticky dough forms.
3. Roll into small balls and refrigerate for 1 hour.

Nutrition Information (per serving):

- Calories: 120
- Protein: 3g
- Carbohydrates: 15g
- Fat: 7g
- Fiber: 3g
- Sugar: 10g
- Portion Size: 2 balls

Baklava-Inspired Yogurt Parfait

Ingredients:

- 1 cup Greek yogurt
- 2 tablespoons crushed walnuts
- 1 tablespoon honey
- 1 tablespoon phyllo dough, crumbled

Instructions:

1. Layer Greek yogurt in a glass.

2. Top with crushed walnuts, drizzle honey, and add crumbled phyllo dough.

3. Repeat the layers and serve.

Nutrition Information (per serving):

- Calories: 220

- Protein: 10g

- Carbohydrates: 15g

- Fat: 15g

- Fiber: 2g

- Sugar: 10g

- Portion Size: 1 serving

Roasted Peach with Cinnamon

Ingredients:

- 2 peaches, halved and pitted

- 1 tablespoon honey

- 1/2 teaspoon cinnamon

Instructions:

1. Preheat oven to 375°F (190°C).
2. Place peach halves on a baking sheet.
3. Drizzle with honey and sprinkle with cinnamon.
4. Roast for 20 minutes, serve warm.

Nutrition Information (per serving):

- Calories: 90
- Protein: 1g
- Carbohydrates: 20g
- Fat: 0.5g
- Fiber: 3g
- Sugar: 15g
- Portion Size: 1 peach half

Lemon Sorbet with Mint

Ingredients:

- 3 cups fresh lemon juice
- 1 cup water
- 1 cup sugar
- 2 tablespoons fresh mint, chopped

Instructions:

1. In a saucepan, combine water and sugar, heat until sugar dissolves.
2. Cool the syrup, then mix with fresh lemon juice.
3. Pour into an ice cream maker and churn according to the manufacturer's instructions.
4. Stir in chopped mint and freeze until firm.

Nutrition Information (per serving):

- Calories: 120
- Protein: 1g
- Carbohydrates: 30g
- Fat: 0.5g
- Fiber: 2g
- Sugar: 25g
- Portion Size: 1/2 cup

Watermelon and Mint Granita

Ingredients:

- 4 cups watermelon, seeded and cubed
- 1/4 cup fresh mint leaves
- 1/4 cup honey

- Juice of 1 lime

Instructions:

1. Blend watermelon, mint, honey, and lime juice until smooth.
2. Pour into a shallow dish and freeze for 3 hours.
3. Scrape with a fork to create a granita texture.

Nutrition Information (per serving):

- Calories: 80
- Protein: 1g
- Carbohydrates: 20g
- Fat: 0.5g
- Fiber: 1g
- Sugar: 18g
- Portion Size: 1/2 cup

Chia Seed Pudding with Pistachios and Dates

Ingredients:

- 1/4 cup chia seeds

- 1 cup almond milk
- 1 tablespoon honey
- 2 tablespoons pistachios, chopped
- 2 tablespoons dates, chopped

Instructions:

1. Mix chia seeds, almond milk, and honey, refrigerate overnight.
2. In the morning, layer with chopped pistachios and dates.

Nutrition Information (per serving):

- Calories: 180
- Protein: 5g
- Carbohydrates: 20g
- Fat: 8g
- Fiber: 8g
- Sugar: 10g
- Portion Size: 1 serving

Orange and Walnut Biscotti

Ingredients:

- 2 cups whole wheat flour
- 1/2 cup honey
- 1/2 cup walnuts, chopped
- Zest of 2 oranges
- 2 eggs
- 1 teaspoon baking powder

Instructions:

1. Preheat oven to 350°F (175°C).
2. Mix whole wheat flour, honey, walnuts, orange zest, eggs, and baking powder.
3. Form into a log, bake for 25-30 minutes.
4. Slice and bake again until crisp.

Nutrition Information (per serving):

- Calories: 160
- Protein: 4g
- Carbohydrates: 20g
- Fat: 8g
- Fiber: 2g

- Sugar: 8g

- Portion Size: 2 biscotti

Fig and Almond Tart

Ingredients:

- 1 sheet puff pastry

- 1 cup almond meal

- 1/4 cup honey

- 6-8 fresh figs, sliced

Instructions:

1. Roll out puff pastry, spread almond meal, and drizzle honey.

2. Arrange fig slices on top.

3. Bake according to puff pastry instructions.

Nutrition Information (per serving):

- Calories: 220

- Protein: 4g

- Carbohydrates: 25g

- Fat: 12g

- Fiber: 3g

- Sugar: 12g
- Portion Size: 1 slice

Chapter 7: Smoothies

Each smoothie is a symphony of flavors and health benefits, combining the richness of natural ingredients. To ensure a delightful experience, we've included not just the recipes but also detailed nutritional information, guiding you towards a wholesome and satisfying treat.

Berry and Spinach Green Smoothie

Ingredients:

- 1 cup mixed berries (strawberries, blueberries, raspberries)
- 1 cup fresh spinach leaves
- 1 banana
- 1/2 cup almond milk
- Ice cubes (optional)

Instructions:

1. Combine berries, spinach, banana, and almond milk in a blender.
2. Blend until smooth.

3. Add ice cubes if desired and blend again.

4. Pour into a glass and enjoy!

Nutrition Information:

- Calories: 150
- Protein: 5g
- Carbohydrates: 30g
- Fat: 2g
- Fiber: 8g
- Sugar: 15g
- Portion Size: 1 serving

Mango and Pineapple Smoothie

Ingredients:

- 1 cup mango chunks (fresh or frozen)
- 1/2 cup pineapple chunks
- 1/2 cup Greek yogurt
- 1/2 cup coconut water
- 1 tablespoon honey

Instructions:

1. Blend mango, pineapple, Greek yogurt, and coconut water until smooth.
2. Add honey and blend again.
3. Pour into a glass and savor the tropical goodness.

Nutrition Information:

- Calories: 180
- Protein: 8g
- Carbohydrates: 35g
- Fat: 3g
- Fiber: 4g
- Sugar: 28g
- Portion Size: 1 serving

Greek Yogurt and Berry Smoothie

Ingredients:

- 1/2 cup mixed berries (blackberries, raspberries, blueberries)
- 1/2 cup Greek yogurt
- 1/2 cup almond milk
- 1 tablespoon chia seeds

- 1 teaspoon honey

Instructions:

1. Blend berries, Greek yogurt, almond milk, and chia seeds until creamy.
2. Add honey and blend briefly.
3. Pour into a glass, and indulge in this protein-packed delight.

Nutrition Information:

- Calories: 200
- Protein: 10g
- Carbohydrates: 25g
- Fat: 6g
- Fiber: 5g
- Sugar: 15g
- Portion Size: 1 serving

Avocado and Kale Smoothie

Ingredients:

- 1/2 ripe avocado
- 1 cup kale leaves, stems removed

- 1/2 banana

- 1 cup coconut water

- 1 tablespoon flaxseeds

Instructions:

1. Blend avocado, kale, banana, and coconut water until silky.

2. Add flaxseeds and blend for an extra nutritional punch.

3. Pour into a glass and relish the creamy goodness.

Nutrition Information:

- Calories: 220

- Protein: 7g

- Carbohydrates: 30g

- Fat: 11g

- Fiber: 8g

- Sugar: 10g

- Portion Size: 1 serving

Mediterranean Citrus Smoothie

Ingredients:

- 1 orange, peeled and segmented
- 1/2 grapefruit, peeled and segmented
- 1/2 cup plain yogurt
- 1 tablespoon honey
- Ice cubes (optional)

Instructions:

1. Blend orange, grapefruit, yogurt, and honey until smooth.
2. Add ice cubes if desired and blend again.
3. Pour into a glass and enjoy the zesty, refreshing taste.

Nutrition Information:

- Calories: 160
- Protein: 5g
- Carbohydrates: 35g
- Fat: 1g
- Fiber: 5g
- Sugar: 25g
- Portion Size: 1 serving

Banana and Almond Butter Smoothie

Ingredients:

- 2 ripe bananas
- 2 tablespoons almond butter
- 1 cup almond milk
- 1/2 teaspoon cinnamon
- 1 tablespoon chia seeds

Instructions:

1. Blend bananas, almond butter, almond milk, and cinnamon until creamy.
2. Add chia seeds and blend briefly.
3. Pour into a glass and revel in the nutty sweetness.

Nutrition Information:

- Calories: 250
- Protein: 8g
- Carbohydrates: 30g
- Fat: 12g
- Fiber: 7g
- Sugar: 15g

- Portion Size: 1 serving

Pomegranate and Blueberry Smoothie

Ingredients:

- 1/2 cup pomegranate seeds
- 1/2 cup blueberries
- 1/2 cup vanilla Greek yogurt
- 1/2 cup coconut water
- 1 tablespoon hemp seeds

Instructions:

1. Blend pomegranate seeds, blueberries, Greek yogurt, and coconut water until luscious.
2. Add hemp seeds and blend for added texture.
3. Pour into a glass and relish the antioxidant-rich goodness.

Nutrition Information:

- Calories: 180
- Protein: 9g

- Carbohydrates: 25g

- Fat: 5g

- Fiber: 6g

- Sugar: 18g

- Portion Size: 1 serving

Spinach and Pineapple Detox Smoothie

Ingredients:

- 1 cup fresh spinach leaves

- 1/2 cup pineapple chunks

- 1/2 cucumber, peeled and sliced

- 1/2 lemon, juiced

- 1 teaspoon ginger, grated

Instructions:

1. Blend spinach, pineapple, cucumber, lemon juice, and ginger until smooth.

2. Pour into a glass and enjoy the detoxifying freshness.

Nutrition Information:

- Calories: 120
- Protein: 4g
- Carbohydrates: 30g
- Fat: 1g
- Fiber: 5g
- Sugar: 15g
- Portion Size: 1 serving

Cucumber and Mint Smoothie

Ingredients:

- 1 cucumber, peeled and sliced
- 1/2 cup fresh mint leaves
- 1/2 cup plain yogurt
- 1 tablespoon honey
- Ice cubes (optional)

Instructions:

1. Blend cucumber, mint, yogurt, and honey until refreshing and smooth.
2. Add ice cubes if desired and blend again.

3. Pour into a glass and savor the cool, invigorating taste.

Nutrition Information:

- Calories: 100
- Protein: 3g
- Carbohydrates: 20g
- Fat: 2g
- Fiber: 3g
- Sugar: 15g
- Portion Size: 1 serving

Turmeric and Ginger Immune-Boosting Smoothie

Ingredients:

- 1 banana
- 1/2 teaspoon turmeric powder
- 1/2 teaspoon grated fresh ginger
- 1 cup orange juice
- 1 tablespoon flaxseeds

Instructions:

1. Blend banana, turmeric, ginger, and orange juice until golden and smooth.
2. Add flaxseeds and blend for an extra health kick.
3. Pour into a glass and enjoy the immune-boosting goodness.

Nutrition Information:

- Calories: 160
- Protein: 4g
- Carbohydrates: 35g
- Fat: 3g
- Fiber: 6g
- Sugar: 20g
- Portion Size: 1 serving

Coconut and Berry Protein Smoothie

Ingredients:

- 1/2 cup mixed berries (strawberries, blueberries, raspberries)
- 1/2 cup coconut milk
- 1/2 cup vanilla protein powder

- 1 tablespoon almond butter

- 1 teaspoon coconut flakes

Instructions:

1. Blend berries, coconut milk, protein powder, and almond butter until creamy.

2. Sprinkle coconut flakes on top for added texture.

3. Pour into a glass and relish the protein-packed delight.

Nutrition Information:

- Calories: 220

- Protein: 15g

- Carbohydrates: 20g

- Fat: 9g

- Fiber: 5g

- Sugar: 10g

- Portion Size: 1 serving

Watermelon and Basil Smoothie

Ingredients:

- 2 cups fresh watermelon, cubed

- 1/2 cup basil leaves
- 1/2 lime, juiced
- 1 tablespoon chia seeds
- Ice cubes (optional)

Instructions:

1. Blend watermelon, basil, lime juice, and chia seeds until smooth.
2. Add ice cubes if desired and blend again.
3. Pour into a glass and enjoy the hydrating and flavorful experience.

Nutrition Information:

- Calories: 120
- Protein: 3g
- Carbohydrates: 25g
- Fat: 2g
- Fiber: 5g
- Sugar: 15g
- Portion Size: 1 serving

Kiwi and Avocado Green Smoothie

Ingredients:

- 2 kiwis, peeled and sliced
- 1/2 ripe avocado
- 1 cup spinach leaves
- 1/2 cup coconut water
- 1 tablespoon honey

Instructions:

1. Blend kiwis, avocado, spinach, coconut water, and honey until velvety.
2. Pour into a glass and relish the green goodness.

Nutrition Information:

- Calories: 180
- Protein: 5g
- Carbohydrates: 30g
- Fat: 8g
- Fiber: 6g
- Sugar: 18g
- Portion Size: 1 serving

Chocolate Avocado Protein Smoothie

Ingredients:

- 1/2 ripe avocado
- 1 tablespoon cocoa powder
- 1/2 cup chocolate protein powder
- 1 cup almond milk
- 1 tablespoon almond butter

Instructions:

1. Blend avocado, cocoa powder, protein powder, almond milk, and almond butter until creamy.
2. Pour into a glass and enjoy the decadent chocolate treat.

Nutrition Information:

- Calories: 240
- Protein: 20g
- Carbohydrates: 20g
- Fat: 10g
- Fiber: 6g
- Sugar: 5g

- Portion Size: 1 serving

Almond and Date Smoothie

Ingredients:

- 1/2 cup almond milk
- 1/2 cup pitted dates
- 1/4 cup almonds
- 1 banana
- 1/2 teaspoon vanilla extract

Instructions:

1. Blend almond milk, dates, almonds, banana, and vanilla extract until smooth.
2. Pour into a glass and savor the naturally sweet and nutty blend.

Nutrition Information:

- Calories: 200
- Protein: 6g
- Carbohydrates: 30g
- Fat: 8g
- Fiber: 5g

- Sugar: 20g
- Portion Size: 1 serving

CONCLUSION

The "Mediterranean Diet Vegetarian Recipes for Type 1 Diabetes," it's evident that managing diabetes can be a delightful journey filled with vibrant flavors and nourishing ingredients. This book is not just a collection of recipes; it's a guide to embracing a lifestyle that harmonizes the principles of the Mediterranean diet with the specific needs of those with Type 1 Diabetes.

Throughout the chapters, we've ventured into the art of crafting balanced and delicious meals that not only cater to the dietary requirements of diabetes management but also celebrate the richness of vegetarian, Mediterranean-inspired cuisine. From hearty breakfasts to satisfying dinners, and from refreshing smoothies to guilt-free desserts, every recipe is a testament to the belief that healthful eating need not compromise on taste.

The 30-day meal plan serves as a practical roadmap, offering a structured approach to incorporate these delectable recipes into your daily life. The diverse array of dishes ensures that monotony is banished from your table, making each meal an exciting and flavorful experience.

More than just a cookbook, this compilation is a companion on your journey towards a healthier and more mindful lifestyle. The Mediterranean diet's emphasis on whole, unprocessed foods, combined with the power of plant-based nutrition, offers not only a means of managing diabetes but also a pathway to overall well-being.

As we close these pages, let it be a reminder that embracing a Mediterranean diet is not a restriction but an invitation to savor the abundance of nature's bounty. Each recipe is crafted with care, inviting you to explore and experiment in the kitchen, turning the act of nourishing your body into a joyful and fulfilling endeavor.

May this book inspire you to approach your meals with creativity, savor every bite with mindfulness, and find pleasure in the journey towards a healthier, diabetes-managing lifestyle. Here's to your well-being, to the joy of cooking, and to a future filled with delicious, diabetes-friendly meals. Cheers to a vibrant and flavorful life!